# 89 Prostate Cancer Juice and Meal Recipes:

## Fight Cancer, Increase Energy, and Feel Healthier Again

By

**Joe Correa CSN**

## COPYRIGHT

## ACKNOWLEDGEMENTS

This book is dedicated to my friends and family that have had mild or serious illnesses so that you may find a solution and make the necessary changes in your life.

# 89 Prostate Cancer Juice and Meal Recipes:

## Fight Cancer, Increase Energy, and Feel Healthier Again

By

**Joe Correa CSN**

# CONTENTS

## ABOUT THE AUTHOR

After years of Research, I honestly believe in the positive effects that proper nutrition can have over the body and mind. My knowledge and experience has helped me live healthier throughout the years and which I have shared with family and friends. The more you know about eating and drinking healthier, the sooner you will want to change your life and eating habits.

Nutrition is a key part in the process of being healthy and living longer so get started today. The first step is the most important and the most significant.

# INTRODUCTION

89 Prostate Cancer Juice and Meal Recipes: Fight Cancer, Increase Energy, and Feel Healthier Again

By Joe Correa CSN

How do you prevent prostate cancer? The answer lies in a proper diet. Our body is a truly incredible organism that has the ability to defend and cure itself. This is why it's crucial to help your immune system to get stronger and boost your overall health.

Eating the right amounts of fruits and vegetables will definitely reduce the risk of prostate cancer. The recommended daily amount of fresh fruits and vegetables is about 4-5 cups. Most people have busy schedules and that is why I definitely believe that juicing is a great option. Combining juicing with healthy meals will give you the best results. Although many kind of fruits and vegetables are extremely healthy, knowing which ones to combine to get the most benefit is the key. Green, red and orange fruits and vegetables are loaded with carotenoids which are especially beneficial for prostate cancer. Some of the best juice and meal ingredients include: spinach, kale, dandelion greens, oranges, grapefruits, berries, carrots, and tomatoes. These tasty fruits and vegetables are the basis of the juice and meal recipes in this book.

To prevent and heal prostate cancer consider these delicious juice and meal recipes that will help you get back on track in a matter of days.

# 89 PROSTATE CANCER JUICE AND MEAL RECIPES: FIGHT CANCER, INCREASE ENERGY, AND FEEL HEALTHIER AGAIN

## JUICES

### 1. Carrot Celery Juice

**Ingredients:**

1 large carrot, sliced

1 large celery, chopped

1 cup of fresh kale, chopped

1 small Granny Smith's apple, cored

1 tbsp of liquid honey

**Preparation:**

Wash and peel the carrot. Cut into thin slices and set aside.

Wash the celery and cut into bite-sized pieces. Set aside.

Rinse the kale under cold running water using a colander. Slightly drain and torn with hands. Set aside.

Wash the apple and cut lengthwise in half. Remove the core and cut into bite-sized pieces. Set aside.

Now, combine carrot, celery, kale, and apple in a juicer and process until juiced. Transfer to a serving glass and stir in the honey.

Add some ice and serve immediately.

**Nutritional information per serving:** Kcal: 179, Protein: 4.6g, Carbs: 34.3g, Fats: 1.1g

## 2. Asparagus Grapefruit Juice

**Ingredients:**

1 cup of asparagus, trimmed and chopped

1 whole grapefruit, peeled

1 whole lime, peeled

1 whole leek, chopped

1 oz of water

**Preparation:**

Wash the asparagus and trim off the woody ends. Chop into small pieces and set aside.

Peel the grapefruit and divide into wedges. Cut each wedge in half and set aside.

Peel the lime and cut lengthwise in half. Set aside.

Wash the leek and cut into bite-sized pieces. Set aside.

Now, combine asparagus, grapefruit, lime, and leek in a juicer and process until well juiced. Transfer to a serving glass and stir in the water.

Add some honey if you like, but it's optional.

Refrigerate for 10 minutes before serving.

Enjoy!

**Nutritional information per serving:** Kcal: 161, Protein: 6.3g, Carbs: 47.7g, Fats: 0.8g

## 3.    Dandelion Juice

**Ingredients:**

1 cup of fresh dandelion greens, torn

2 medium-sized celery stalks, chopped

1 whole lemon, peeled

1 small Granny Smith's apple, cored

1 cup of cucumber, sliced

**Preparation:**

Wash dandelion greens thoroughly and torn with hands into small pieces. Set aside.

Wash the celery and cut into bite-sized pieces. Set aside.

Peel the lemon and cut lengthwise in half. Set aside.

Wash the apple and cut in half. Remove the core and cut into bite-sized pieces. Set aside.

Wash the cucumber and cut into thin slices. Fill the measuring cup and reserve the rest for later.

Now, combine dandelions, celery, lemon, apple, and cucumber in a juicer and process until juiced.

Transfer to a serving glass and add some crushed ice before serving.

**Nutritional information per serving:** Kcal: 97, Protein: 2.9g, Carbs: 29.7g, Fats: 0.7g

## 4.  Broccoli Banana Juice

**Ingredients:**

1 cup of broccoli, chopped

1 large banana, sliced

1 small green apple, cored

1 small ginger knob, peeled

1 tbsp of liquid honey

**Preparation:**

Wash the broccoli and trim off the outer layers. Cut into small pieces and fill the measuring cup. Reserve the rest for later.

Peel the banana and cut into small slices. Set aside.

Wash the apple and cut in half. Remove the core and cut into bite-sized pieces. Set aside.

Peel the ginger knob and set aside.

Now, combine broccoli, banana, apple, and ginger in a juicer and process until well juiced. Transfer to a serving glass and stir in the honey.

Refrigerate for 10 minutes before serving.

**Nutritional information per serving:** Kcal: 261, Protein: 4.8g, Carbs: 57.7g, Fats: 1.1g

## 5.     Green Tea Juice

**Ingredients:**

1 tsp of green tea

2 tbsp of hot water

2 whole kiwis, peeled

1 medium-sized pear, chopped

1 cup of fresh spinach, torn

1 cup of fresh mint, roughly chopped

1 whole lime, peeled

**Preparation:**

Combine green tea and hot water in a small bowl. Stir well and set aside to soak for 3 minutes.

Peel the kiwis and cut lengthwise in half. Set aside.

Wash the pear and remove the core. Cut into bite-sized pieces and set aside.

Wash the spinach under cold running water using a colander. Torn with hands and set aside.

Wash the mint and roughly chop it. Fill the measuring cup and reserve the rest for later.

Peel the lime and cut lengthwise in half. Set aside.

Now, combine green tea mixture, kiwis, pear, spinach, mint, and lime in a juicer and process until juiced. Transfer to a serving glass and add some ice before serving.

Enjoy!

**Nutritional information per serving:** Kcal: 195, Protein: 9.4g, Carbs: 62.4g, Fats: 2.1g

## 6.     Pomegranate Asparagus Juice

**Ingredients:**

1 cup of pomegranate seeds

1 cup of fresh asparagus, trimmed and chopped

1 whole lemon, peeled

1 tbsp of liquid honey

1 oz of water

**Preparation:**

Cut the top of the pomegranate fruit using a sharp paring knife. Slice down to each of the white membranes inside of the fruit. Pop the seeds into a measuring cup and set aside.

Wash the asparagus and trim off the woody ends. Cut into bite-sized pieces and set aside.

Peel the lemon and cut into quarters. Set aside.

Now, combine pomegranate seeds, asparagus, and lemon in a juicer and process until well juiced. Transfer to a serving glass and stir in the honey and water.

Add some ice and enjoy!

**Nutritional information per serving:** Kcal: 145, Protein: 5.1g, Carbs: 26.8g, Fats: 1.3g

## 7.　　Spinach Tomato Juice

**Ingredients:**

1 cup of fresh spinach, chopped

6 cherry tomatoes, halved

1 cup of cucumber, sliced

1 small ginger knob, peeled

¼ tsp of salt

**Preparation:**

Wash the spinach thoroughly under cold running water. Slightly drain and chop into small pieces. Set aside.

Wash the cherry tomatoes and remove the stems. Cut each tomato in half and set aside.

Wash the cucumber and cut into thin slices. Fill the measuring cup and reserve the rest for later.

Now, combine spinach, tomatoes, cucumber, and ginger in a juicer and process until juiced. Transfer to a serving glass and stir in the salt.

Serve immediately.

**Nutritional information per serving:** Kcal: 52, Protein: 7.4g, Carbs: 14.5g, Fats: 1.1g

## 8.     Watermelon Blueberry Juice

**Ingredients:**

1 cup of watermelon, cubed

2 cups of blueberries

1 whole lime, peeled

1 cup of fresh basil, torn

¼ tsp of cayenne pepper, ground

1 oz of water

**Preparation:**

Cut one large watermelon wedge. Using a sharp paring knife, peel and cut into small cubes. Remove the seeds and set aside.

Place the blueberries in a large colander. Rinse well under cold running water and set aside.

Peel the lime and cut lengthwise in half. Set aside.

Wash the basil and roughly torn it with hands. Set aside.

Now, combine watermelon, blueberries, lime, and basil in a juicer. Process until juiced. Transfer to a serving glass and stir in the cayenne pepper and water.

Refrigerate for 10 minutes before serving.

**Nutritional information per serving:** Kcal: 198, Protein: 4.1g, Carbs: 58.7g, Fats: 1.4g

## 9.    Carrot Plum Juice

**Ingredients:**

1 cup of baby carrots, sliced

4 whole plum, chopped

1 cup of Romaine lettuce, shredded

1 cup of mustard greens, torn

1 oz of water

**Preparation:**

Wash and peel the carrots. Cut into thin slices and fill the measuring cup. Reserve the rest in the refrigerator.

Wash the plums and cut each in half. Remove the pits and set aside.

Combine lettuce and mustard greens in a large colander. Rinse well under cold running water. Shred the lettuce torn the mustard greens using hands. Set aside.

Now, combine carrots, plums, lettuce, and mustard greens in a juicer and process until juiced. Transfer to a serving glass and stir in the water.

Serve cold.

**Nutritional information per serving:** Kcal: 128, Protein: 4.8g, Carbs: 39.1g, Fats: 1.3g

## 10.  Pepper Avocado Juice

**Ingredients:**

2 medium-sized red bell peppers, chopped

1 cup of avocado, sliced

1 cup of purple cabbage, chopped

1 whole leek, chopped

1 whole lime, peeled

**Preparation:**

Wash the peppers and cut in half. Remove the seeds and cut into small pieces. Set aside.

Peel the avocado and cut lengthwise in half. Cut into thin slices and reserve the rest in the refrigerator. Set aside.

Wash the cabbage thoroughly and chop into small pieces. Set aside.

Wash the leek and cut into bite-sized pieces. Set aside.

Peel the lime and cut lengthwise in half. Set aside.

Now, combine peppers, avocado, cabbage, leek, and lime in a juicer and process until juiced. Transfer to a serving glass and refrigerate for 15 minutes before serving.

Enjoy!

**Nutritional information per serving:** Kcal: 327, Protein: 8.1g, Carbs: 49.6g, Fats: 22.5g

## 11.   Grapefruit Mango Juice

**Ingredients:**

1 whole grapefruit, peeled

1 cup of mango, cut into chunks

1 cup of fresh mint, roughly chopped

1 large banana, peeled

2 large strawberries, chopped

**Preparation:**

Peel the grapefruit and divide into wedges. Cut each wedge in half and set aside.

Peel the mango and cut into small chunks. Fill the measuring cup and reserve the rest in the refrigerator. Set aside.

Wash the mint roughly and torn with hands. Set aside.

Peel the banana and cut into small pieces. Set aside.

Wash the strawberries and remove the stems. Cut into bite-sized pieces and set aside.

Now, combine grapefruit, mango, mint, banana, and strawberries in a juicer and process until juiced. Transfer to a serving glass and add some ice cubes before serving.

Enjoy!

**Nutritional information per serving:** Kcal: 301, Protein: 5.9g, Carbs: 88.5g, Fats: 1.7g

## 12.    Beet Lemon Juice

**Ingredients:**

1 whole beet, sliced

1 whole lemon, peeled

1 cup of cucumber, sliced

1 medium-sized orange, peeled

1 tbsp of liquid honey

**Preparation:**

Wash the beet and trim off the green parts. Cut into thin slices and set aside.

Peel the lemon and cut into quarters. Set aside.

Wash the cucumber and cut into thin slices. Fill the measuring cup and reserve the rest in the refrigerator.

Peel the orange and divide into wedges. Cut each wedge in half and set aside.

Now, combine beet, lemon, cucumber, and orange in a juicer and process until juiced. Transfer to a serving glass and stir in the honey.

Add some ice and serve immediately.

**Nutritional information per serving:** Kcal: 154, Protein: 3.5g, Carbs: 30.5g, Fats: 0.5g

## 13.    Green Bean Juice

**Ingredients:**

1 cup of green beans, chopped

1 medium-sized Granny Smith's apple, cored

1 medium-sized celery stalk, cut into bite-sized pieces

1 cup of fresh spinach, chopped

**Preparation:**

Wash the green beans and chop into bite-sized pieces. Fill the measuring cup and reserve the rest for later.

Wash the apple and cut in half. Remove the core and cut into small chunks. Set aside.

Wash the celery and cut into bite-sized pieces. Set aside.

Wash the spinach thoroughly under cold running water. Chop into small pieces and fill the measuring cup. Reserve the rest for later.

Now, combine green beans, apple, celery, and spinach in a juicer and process until well juiced. Transfer to serving glass and add some ice before serving.

Enjoy!

**Nutritional information per serving:** Kcal: 140, Protein: 8.5g, Carbs: 37.3g, Fats: 1.4g

## 14.    Pepper Kale Juice

**Ingredients:**

1 medium-sized red bell pepper, chopped

1 cup of fresh kale, chopped

1 cup of parsley, torn

1 large celery stalk, chopped

1 cup of cucumber, sliced

1 oz of water

**Preparation:**

Wash the bell pepper and cut lengthwise in half. Scrape out the seeds and remove the stem. Cut into bite-sized pieces and set aside.

Wash the kale thoroughly under cold running water. Slightly drain and chop it into small pieces. Set aside.

Wash the parsley and torn with hands. Fill the measuring cup and reserve the rest for later.

Wash the celery stalk and chop it into bite-sized pieces. Set aside.

Wash the cucumber and cut into thin slices. Fill the measuring cup and reserve the rest for later.

Now, combine bell pepper, kale, parsley, celery, and cucumber in a juicer and process until juiced. Transfer to a serving glass and stir in the water. Add some ice and serve immediately.

Enjoy!

**Nutritional information per serving:** Kcal: 77, Protein: 6.6g, Carbs: 20.6g, Fats: 1.6g

## 15.   Basil Zucchini Juice

**Ingredients:**

1 cup of fresh basil, chopped

1 medium-sized zucchini, sliced

1 whole lemon, peeled

1 whole lime, peeled

1 oz of water

**Preparation:**

Wash the basil thoroughly under cold running water. Slightly drain and chop into small pieces. Set aside.

Wash the zucchini and cut into thin slices. Set aside.

Peel the lemon and lime. Cut each fruit into quarters and set aside.

Now, combine basil, zucchini, lemon, and lime in a juicer. Process until well juiced. Transfer to a serving glass and stir in the water.

Refrigerate for 10 minutes before serving.

**Nutritional information per serving:** Kcal: 50, Protein: 3.9g, Carbs: 15.8g, Fats: 0.9g

## 16.    Blueberry Grape Juice

**Ingredients:**

1 cup of blueberries

1 cup of black grapes

1 small Golden Delicious apple, cored

¼ tsp of cinnamon, ground

**Preparation:**

Wash the blueberries using a colander. Slightly drain and set aside.

Wash the grapes and fill the measuring cup. Reserve the rest for later.

Wash the apple and cut in half. Remove the core and cut into bite-sized pieces. Set aside.

Now, combine blueberries, grapes, and apple in a juicer and process until juiced. Transfer to a serving glass and stir in the cinnamon.

Add some ice before serving and enjoy!

**Nutritional information per serving:** Kcal: 191, Protein: 2.1g, Carbs: 54.7g, Fats: 1g

## 17.    Mango Raspberry Juice

**Ingredients:**

1 cup of mango, chunked

1 cup of raspberries

1 small peach, pitted

3 whole apricots, chopped

**Preparation:**

Peel the mango and cut into small chunks. Fill the measuring cup and reserve the rest for later.

Wash the raspberries using a colander. Slightly drain and fill the measuring cup. Reserve the rest in the refrigerator or freezer for later.

Wash the peach and cut in half. Remove the pit and cut into bite-sized pieces. Set aside.

Wash the apricots and cut in half. Remove the pits and cut in quarters. Set aside.

Now, combine mango, raspberries, peach, and apricots in a juicer and process until juiced. Transfer to a serving glass refrigerate for 10 minutes before serving.

You can garnish with some fresh mint if you like, but it's optional.

**Nutritional information per serving:** Kcal: 206, Protein: 5.5g, Carbs: 63.5g, Fats: 2.1g

## 18.    Pineapple Beet Juice

**Ingredients:**

1 cup of pineapple, chunked

1 whole beet, sliced

1 small orange, wedged

2 tbsp of coconut water

¼ tsp of ginger, ground

**Preparation:**

Cut the top of a pineapple and peel it using a sharp paring knife. Cut into small chunks and fill the measuring cup. Reserve the rest of the pineapple in a refrigerator.

Wash and trim off the beet. Cut into small slices and set aside.

Peel the orange and divide into wedges. Cut each wedge in half and set aside.

Now, combine pineapple, beet, and orange in a juicer and process until juiced. Transfer to a serving glass and stir in the coconut water and ginger.

Add some crushed ice and serve immediately.

**Nutritional information per serving:** Kcal: 135, Protein: 3.1g, Carbs: 40.7g, Fats: 0.5g

## 19.    Kiwi Banana Juice

**Ingredients:**

3 whole kiwis, peeled

1 large banana, chopped

1 large strawberry, chopped

1 small apple, cored

¼ tsp of cinnamon, ground

**Preparation:**

Peel the kiwis and cut lengthwise in half. Set aside.

Peel the banana and chop into small chunks. Set aside.

Wash the strawberry and remove the stem. Cut into small pieces and set aside.

Wash the apple and cut in half. Remove the core and cut into bite-sized pieces. Set aside.

Now, combine kiwis, banana, strawberry, and apple in a juicer and process until juiced. Transfer to a serving glass and stir in the cinnamon.

Refrigerate for 10 minutes before serving.

Enjoy!

**Nutritional information per serving:** Kcal: 292, Protein: 4.4g, Carbs: 85g, Fats: 1.9g

## 20.  Avocado Lemon Juice

**Ingredients:**

1 cup of avocado, cubed

1 whole lemon, peeled

1 cup of cranberries

1 cup of cucumber, sliced

1 cup of cherries, pitted

**Preparation:**

Peel the avocado and cut into small cubes. Fill the measuring cup and reserve the rest in the refrigerator. Set aside.

Peel the lemon and cut lengthwise in half. Set aside.

Wash the cranberries and set aside.

Wash the cucumber and cut into slices. Fill the measuring cup and reserve the  the rest for later.

Wash the cherries and cut each in half. Remove the pits and set aside.

Now, combine avocado, cranberries, cucumber, and cherries in a juicer and process until juiced. Transfer to a serving glass and add some ice before serving.

Enjoy!

**Nutritional information per serving:** Kcal: 321, Protein: 5.8g, Carbs: 54.4g, Fats: 22.6g

## 21.    Pomegranate Blackberry Juice

**Ingredients:**

1 cup of pomegranate seeds

1 cup of blackberries

1 whole lemon, peeled

1 medium-sized carrot, sliced

1 oz of water

**Preparation:**

Cut the top of the pomegranate fruit using a sharp paring knife. Slice down to each of the white membranes inside of the fruit. Pop the seeds into a measuring cup and set aside.

Wash the blackberries using a colander. Fill the measuring cup and reserve the rest. Set aside.

Peel the lemon and cut lengthwise in half. Set aside.

Wash and peel the carrot. Cut into thin slices and set aside.

Now, combine pomegranate seeds, blackberries, lemon, and carrot in a juicer. Process until juiced and transfer to a serving glass.

Add some ice or refrigerate for a while before serving.

**Nutritional information per serving:** Kcal: 119, Protein: 4.6g, Carbs: 41.3g, Fats: 2.1g

## 22.    Celery Kale Juice

**Ingredients:**

1 cup of celery, chopped

1 cup of fresh kale, torn

1 cup of fresh mint, torn

1 whole lime, peeled

1 small Granny Smith's apple, cored

**Preparation:**

Wash the celery and chop into small pieces. Fill the measuring cup and set aside.

Combine kale and mint in a large colander. Wash thoroughly under cold running water. Slightly drain and torn with hands. Set aside.

Peel the lime and cut into small pieces. Set aside.

Wash the apple and cut in half. Remove the core and cut into bite-sized pieces. Set aside.

Now, combine celery, kale, mint, lime, and apple in a juicer and process until juiced. Transfer to a serving glass and add some ice before serving.

Enjoy!

**Nutritional information per serving:** Kcal: 121, Protein: 5.3g, Carbs: 35.8g, Fats: 1.3g

## 23.    Potato Zucchini Juice

**Ingredients:**

1 cup of sweet potatoes, cubed

1 small zucchini, sliced

1 small apple, cored

¼ tsp of ginger, ground

**Preparation:**

Peel the sweet potato and cut into small cubes. Fill the measuring cup and reserve the rest for later.

Peel the zucchini and cut into thin slices. Set aside.

Wash the apple and cut in half. Remove the core and cut into bite-sized pieces. Set aside.

Now, combine sweet potatoes, zucchini, and apple in a juicer. Process until well juiced. Transfer to a serving glass and stir in the ginger.

Refrigerate for 10 minutes before serving.

Enjoy!

**Nutritional information per serving:** Kcal: 181, Protein: 4.2g, Carbs: 50.1g, Fats: 0.7g

## 24.    Apricot Plum Juice

**Ingredients:**

2 whole apricots, pitted

2 whole plums, chopped

1 cup of cherries, pitted

1 small orange, peeled

1 tbsp of coconut water

**Preparation:**

Wash the apricots and cut in half. Remove the pits and cut all into small pieces. Set aside.

Wash the plums and cut in half. Remove the pits and cut into bite-sized pieces. Set aside.

Wash the cherries using a colander. Remove the pits and set aside.

Peel the orange and divide into wedges. Cut each wedge in half and set aside.

Now, combine apricots, plums, cherries, and orange in a juicer and process until well juiced. Transfer to a serving glass and stir in the coconut water.

Refrigerate for 10 minutes before serving.

Enjoy!

**Nutritional information per serving:** Kcal: 191, Protein: 4.3g, Carbs: 56.3g, Fats: 1.1g

## 25.    Fennel Broccoli Juice

**Ingredients:**

1 cup of fennel, chopped

1 cup of broccoli, chopped

1 cup of Brussels sprouts, halved

1 cup of watercress, torn

1 cup of cucumber, sliced

**Preparation:**

Wash the fennel and trim off the outer leaves. Using  a sharp paring knife, cut into small pieces and fill the measuring cup. Reserve the rest for later.

Wash the broccoli and cut into small pieces. Fill the measuring cup and reserve the rest in the refrigerator. Set aside.

Wash the Brussels sprouts and trim off the outer layers. Cut in half and set aside.

Wash the watercress thoroughly under cold running water. Slightly drain and torn with hands. Set aside.

Wash the cucumber and cut into thin slices. Fill the measuring cup and reserve the rest for later.

Now, combine fennel, broccoli, Brussels sprouts, watercress, and cucumber in a juicer and process until juiced. Transfer to a serving glass and refrigerate for 10 minutes before serving.

Enjoy!

**Nutritional information per serving:** Kcal: 72, Protein: 7.7g, Carbs: 22.6g, Fats: 0.8g

## 26.　　**Cranberry Pear Juice**

**Ingredients:**

1 cup of cranberries

1 medium-sized pear, chopped

1 whole lemon, peeled

½ cup of strawberries, sliced

1 small ginger knob, peeled

1 oz of water

**Preparation:**

Wash the cranberries and fill the measuring cup. Set aside.

Wash the pear and cut in half. Remove the core and cut into small pieces. Set aside.

Peel the lemon and cut in half. Set aside.

Wash the strawberries and remove the stems. Cut into small pieces and fill the measuring cup. Set aside.

Peel the ginger knob and set aside.

Now, combine cranberries, pear, lemon, strawberries, and ginger in a juicer and process until juiced. Transfer to a serving glass and stir in the water.

Serve cold.

**Nutritional information per serving:** Kcal: 143, Protein: 2.4g, Carbs: 52.7g, Fats: 0.8g

## 27.    Beet Green Carrot Juice

**Ingredients:**

1 cup of beet greens, torn

1 large carrot, sliced

1 medium-sized orange, peeled

1 cup of cantaloupe, chopped

¼ tsp of ginger, ground

**Preparation:**

Wash the beet greens thoroughly under cold running water. Drain and torn with hands. Set aside.

Wash the carrot and cut into thin slices. Set aside.

Peel the orange and divide into wedges. Cut each wedge in half and set aside.

Cut the cantaloupe in half. Scoop out the seeds and cut one large wedge. Peel it and cut into small pieces. Fill the measuring cup and reserve the rest of the cantaloupe in a refrigerator.

Now, combine beet greens, carrot, orange, and cantaloupe in a juicer and process until juiced. Transfer to a serving glass and stir in the ginger.

Serve cold.

**Nutritional information per serving:** Kcal: 99, Protein: 3.5g, Carbs: 30.5g, Fats: 0.6g

## 28.    Collard Greens Cucumber Juice

**Ingredients:**

2 cups of collard greens, chopped

1 cup of cucumber, sliced

1 whole lime, peeled

1 cup of Swiss chard, chopped

1 large celery stalk, chopped

1 oz of water

¼ tsp of salt

**Preparation:**

Combine collard greens and Swiss chard in a large colander. Wash it under running water and slightly drain. Chop into small pieces and set aside.

Wash the cucumber and cut into thin slices. Fill the measuring cup and reserve the rest in the refrigerator.

Peel the lime and cut lengthwise in half. Set aside.

Wash the celery and cut into small pieces. Set aside.

Now, combine collard greens, cucumber, lime, Swiss chard, and celery in a juicer and process until juiced. Transfer to a serving glass and stir in the water and salt. Refrigerate for 10 minutes before serving.

Enjoy!

**Nutritional information per serving:** Kcal: 40, Protein: 3.8g, Carbs: 12.7g, Fats: 0.7g

## 29.   Pumpkin Pepper Juice

**Ingredients:**

1 cup of pumpkin, cubed

1 large yellow bell pepper, chopped

1 small zucchini, sliced

¼ tsp of cinnamon, ground

**Preparation:**

Cut the pumpkin lengthwise in half. Scoop out the seeds and cut one large wedge. Peel it and fill the measuring cup. Wrap the rest of the pumpkin in a plastic foil and refrigerate for later.

Wash the bell pepper and cut in half. Remove the seeds and stem. Cut into bite-sized pieces and set aside.

Wash the zucchini thoroughly and cut into thin slices. Set aside.

Now, combine pumpkin, bell pepper, and zucchini in a juicer and process until juiced. Transfer to a serving glass and stir in the cinnamon.

Refrigerate for 10 minutes before serving.

Enjoy!

**Nutritional information per serving:** Kcal: 86, Protein: 4.5g, Carbs: 22.9g, Fats: 0.9g

## 30.    Kale Celery Juice

**Ingredients:**

1 cup of fresh kale, chopped

2 medium-sized celery stalk, chopped

1 small apple, cored

1 cup of Romaine lettuce, shredded

**Preparation:**

Wash the kale thoroughly under cold running water. Slightly drain and chop it into small pieces. Set aside.

Wash the celery stalks and cut into bite-sized pieces. Set aside.

Wash the apple and cut in half. remove the core and cut into small pieces. Set aside.

Wash the lettuce leaves and shred it. Fill the measuring cup and reserve the rest for later.

Now, combine kale, celery, apple, and lettuce in a juicer and process until juiced. Transfer to a serving glass and add some ice before serving.

Enjoy!

**Nutritional information per serving:** Kcal: 103, Protein: 4.6g, Carbs: 29.4g, Fats: 1.2g

## 31.    Melon Lime Juice

**Ingredients:**

1 medium-sized wedge of honeydew melon

1 whole lime, peeled

1 small Granny Smith's apple, cored

1 large banana, peeled

¼ tsp of cinnamon, ground

**Preparation:**

Cut one large honeydew melon wedge and peel it. Remove the seeds and cut into bite-sized pieces. Wrap the rest of the melon in a plastic foil and refrigerate.

Peel the lime and cut lengthwise in half. Set aside.

Wash the apple and cut in half. Remove the core and cut into bite-sized pieces. Set aside.

Peel the banana and chop into small chunks. Set aside.

Now, combine melon, lime, apple, and banana in a juicer and process until juiced. Transfer to a serving glass and stir in the cinnamon.

Refrigerate for 10 minutes before serving.

**Nutritional information per serving:** Kcal: 226, Protein: 4.6g, Carbs: 29.4g, Fats: 1.2g

## 32.　　Guava Cherry Juice

**Ingredients:**

1 whole guava, peeled

1 cup of cherries, pitted

1 medium-sized orange, wedged

1 whole apricot, pitted

**Preparation:**

Peel the guava and cut into small chunks. Set aside.

Wash the cherries using a colander. Remove the stems and cut each in half. Remove the pits and fill the measuring cup. Set aside.

Peel the orange and divide into wedges. Cut each wedge in half and set aside.

Wash the apricot and cut in half. Remove the pit and cut into bite-sized pieces. Set aside.

Now, combine guava, cherries, orange, and apricot in a juicer and process until juiced. Transfer to a serving glass and add some ice.

Serve immediately.

**Nutritional information per serving:** Kcal: 173, Protein: 4.7g, Carbs: 51.8g, Fats: 1.1g

## 33.  Mango Kiwi Juice

**Ingredients:**

1 cup of mango, chunked

1 whole kiwi, peeled

1 cup of fresh spinach, chopped

1 small ginger knob, peeled

2 tbsp of coconut water

**Preparation:**

Peel the mango and cut into small chunks. Fill the measuring cup and reserve the rest in the refrigerator.

Peel the kiwi and cut lengthwise in half. Set aside.

Wash the spinach thoroughly under cold running water. Slightly drain and chop it into small pieces. Set aside.

Peel the ginger knob and set aside.

Now, combine mango, kiwi, spinach, and ginger in a juicer and process until juiced. Transfer to a serving glass and stir in the coconut water. Refrigerate for 10 minutes before serving.

Enjoy!

**Nutritional information per serving:** Kcal: 190, Protein: 9.1g, Carbs: 53.6g, Fats: 2.2g

## 34.    Pomegranate Plum Juice

**Ingredients:**

1 cup of pomegranate seeds

2 whole plums, pitted

1 small Golden Delicious apple, cored

1 large strawberry, chopped

**Preparation:**

Cut the top of the pomegranate fruit using a sharp paring knife. Slice down to each of the white membranes inside of the fruit. Pop the seeds into a measuring cup and set aside.

Wash the plums and cut lengthwise in half. Remove the pits and cut into small pieces. Set aside.

Wash the apple and cut in half. Remove the core and cut into bite-sized pieces. Set aside.

Wash the strawberry and remove the stem. Cut into small pieces and set aside.

Now, combine pomegranate seeds, plums, apple, and strawberry in a juicer and process until juiced. Transfer to a serving glass and add some crushed ice.

Serve immediately.

**Nutritional information per serving:** Kcal: 176, Protein: 2.8g, Carbs: 50.3g, Fats: 1.6g

## 35.    Watermelon Cranberry Juice

**Ingredients:**

1 cup of watermelon, chopped

1 cup of whole cranberries

1 whole lemon, peeled

1 cup of fresh mint, chopped

1 tbsp of liquid honey

**Preparation:**

Cut the watermelon lengthwise. For one cup, you will need a large slice. Peel and cut into chunks. Remove the seeds and set aside. Reserve the rest for some other juices.

Wash the cranberries using a colander. Fill the measuring cup and reserve the rest in the refrigerator.

Peel the lemon and cut lengthwise in half. Set aside.

Wash the mint thoroughly under cold running water and roughly chop it. Set aside.

Now, combine watermelon, cranberries, lemon, and mint in a juicer and process until juiced. Transfer to a serving glass and stir in the honey.

Add few ice cubes and serve immediately.

Enjoy!

**Nutritional information per serving:** Kcal: 93, Protein: 2.9g, Carbs: 32.8g, Fats: 0.7g

## 36.    Grape Pineapple Juice

**Ingredients:**

1 cup of black grapes

1 cup of pineapple, chunked

1 tsp of vanilla extract

**Preparation:**

In a heavy-bottomed pot, combine grapes and one cup of water. Bring it to a boil over a medium-high temperature, stirring occasionally. Stir in the vanilla extract and remove from the heat. Set aside to cool completely.

Cut the top of a pineapple fruit. Using a sharp paring knife, peel it and cut into thin slices. Fill the measuring cup and reserve the rest for later.

Now, combine grape mixture and pineapple in a juicer and process until well juiced. Transfer to a serving glass and refrigerate for 20 minutes before serving.

Garnish with some fresh mint, but it's optional.

Enjoy!

**Nutritional information per serving:** Kcal: 200, Protein: 2.1g, Carbs: 57g, Fats: 0.8g

## 37.    Tomato Celery Juice

**Ingredients:**

5 cherry tomatoes, halved

1 large celery stalk, chopped

1 cup of cucumber, sliced

1 cup of fresh parsley, chopped

¼ tsp of salt

¼ tsp of black pepper, ground

½ tsp of Tabasco sauce

1 oz of water

**Preparation:**

Wash the cherry tomatoes and remove the stems. Cut each tomato in half and set aside.

Wash the celery stalk and chop it into bite-sized pieces. Set aside.

Wash the cucumber and cut into thin slices. Fill the measuring cup and reserve the rest for later.

Place the parsley in a colander and rinse it thoroughly. Slightly drain and chop into small pieces. Set aside.

Now, combine cherry tomatoes, celery, cucumber, and parsley in a juicer and process until juiced. Transfer to a serving glass and stir in the salt, pepper, Tabasco sauce, and water.

Serve immediately!

**Nutritional information per serving:** Kcal: 38, Protein: 3.3g, Carbs: 10.9g, Fats: 0.8g

## 38.    Blueberry Ginger Juice

**Ingredients:**

2 cups of blueberries

1 small ginger knob, peeled and chopped

1 medium-sized blood orange, peeled

1 cup of black grapes

**Preparation:**

Place the blueberries in a colander. Wash thoroughly under cold running water and drain. Fill the measuring cups and reserve the rest in the freezer.

Peel the ginger and cut into small pieces. Set aside.

Peel the orange and divide into wedges. Cut each wedge in half and set aside.

Wash the grapes and fill the measuring cup. Set aside.

Now, combine blueberries, ginger, orange, and grapes in a juicer and process until juiced. Transfer to a serving glass and add few ice cubes before serving.

Enjoy!

**Nutritional information per serving:** Kcal: 254, Protein: 4.1g, Carbs: 75.2g, Fats: 1.5g

## 39.    Avocado Papaya Juice

**Ingredients:**

1 cup of avocado, cubed

1 small papaya, chopped

1 cup of cherries, halved

1 whole lemon, peeled

¼ tsp of cinnamon, ground

1 oz of water

**Preparation:**

Peel the avocado and cut lengthwise in half. Remove the pit and cut into small cubes. Fill the measuring cup and reserve the rest for later.

Peel the papaya and cut into small chunks. Set aside.

Peel the lemon and cut lengthwise in half. Set aside.

Now, combine avocado, papaya, and lemon in a juicer and process until juiced. Transfer to a serving glass and stir in the cinnamon and water.

Refrigerate for 15 minutes before serving and enjoy!

**Nutritional information per serving:** Kcal: 343, Protein: 5.8g, Carbs: 57.3g, Fats: 22.8g

## 40.    Pumpkin Apple Juice

### Ingredients:

1 cup of pumpkin, cubed

1 small Granny Smith's apple, cored

1 medium-sized carrot, sliced

1 cup of cucumber, sliced

¼ tsp of cinnamon, ground

¼ tsp of ginger, ground

### Preparation:

Cut the pumpkin in half and scoop out the seeds. Wash it and cut one large wedge. Peel it and cut into small cubes. Fill the measuring cup and reserve the rest in the refrigerator.

Wash the apple and cut lengthwise in half. Remove the core and cut into small pieces. Set aside.

Wash and peel the carrot. Cut into thin slices and set aside.

Wash the cucumber and cut into thin slices. Fill the measuring cup and reserve the rest for later.

Now, combine pumpkin, apple, carrot, and cucumber in a juicer and process until juiced. Transfer to a serving glass and stir in the cinnamon and ginger.

Refrigerate for 10 minutes before serving.

**Nutritional information per serving:** Kcal: 121, Protein: 2.7g, Carbs: 34.8g, Fats: 0.6g

## 41.    Peach Lime Juice

**Ingredients:**

2 large peaches, pitted

1 whole lime, peeled

1 cup of apricots, sliced

1 large banana, peeled

**Preparation:**

Wash the peaches and cut in half. Remove the pits and cut each half into bite-sized pieces. Set aside.

Peel the lime and roughly chop it. Make sure to reserve lime juice while cutting.

Wash the apricots and cut in half. Remove the pits and cut into small pieces. Fill the measuring cup and set aside.

Peel the banana and cut into small chunks. Set aside.

Now, combine peaches, lime, apricots, and banana in a juicer and process until juiced. Transfer to a serving glass and add some crushed ice before serving.

Enjoy!

**Nutritional information per serving:** Kcal: 299, Protein: 7.2g, Carbs: 86.5g, Fats: 2g

## 42.  Artichoke Spinach Juice

**Ingredients:**

1 medium-sized artichoke, chopped

1 cup of fresh spinach, chopped

1 cup of green beans, chopped

1 small green bell pepper, sliced

1 small ginger knob, peeled and sliced

**Preparation:**

Trim off the outer leaves of the artichoke using a sharp paring knife. Wash it and cut into bite-sized pieces. Set aside.

Using a colander, rinse the spinach thoroughly under cold running water. Chop into small pieces and set aside.

Place the beans in a deep pot. Add 1 cup of water and bring it to a boil. Cook for 5 minutes and remove from the heat. Set aside to cool completely.

Wash the bell pepper and cut in half. Remove the seeds and stem. Cut into small rings and set aside.

Peel the ginger knob and chop it into small pieces. Set aside.

Now, combine artichoke, spinach, green beans, bell pepper, and ginger in a juicer and process until juiced. Transfer to a serving glass and refrigerate for 10 minutes before serving.

**Nutritional information per serving:** Kcal: 95, Protein: 11.9g, Carbs: 29.4g, Fats: 1.3g

## 43.    Orange Pear Juice

**Ingredients:**

1 medium-sized orange, peeled

1 medium-sized pear, chopped

1 whole plum, pitted

1 whole lemon, peeled

1 oz of water

**Preparation:**

Peel the orange and divide into wedges. Cut each wedge in half and set aside.

Wash the pear and cut in half. Remove the core and chop into small pieces. Set aside.

Wash the plum and cut in half. Remove the pit and cut in small pieces.

Peel the lemon and cut into quarters. Set aside.

Now, combine orange, pear, plum, and lemon in a juicer and process until juiced. Transfer to a serving glass and stir in the water.

You can add a pinch of minced mint for some extra smooth flavor, but it's optional.

Add some crushed ice and serve immediately.

**Nutritional information per serving:** Kcal: 166, Protein: 2.9g, Carbs: 55.4g, Fats: 0.8g

## 44.    Carrot Grapefruit Juice

**Ingredients:**

2 medium-sized carrots, sliced

1 whole grapefruit, wedged

1 cup of Romaine lettuce, shredded

1 cup of fresh mint, chopped

1 whole lime, peeled

**Preparation:**

Wash and peel the carrots. Cut into thin slices and set aside.

Peel the grapefruit and divide into wedges. Cut each wedge in half and set aside.

Wash the lettuce thoroughly under cold running water. Shred it and fill the measuring cup. Reserve the rest for later.

Wash the mint and then place it in a medium bowl. Add one cup of hot water and let it soak for 10 minutes. Slightly drain and set aside.

Peel the lime and cut lengthwise in half. Set aside.

Now, combine carrots, grapefruit, lettuce, mint, and lime in a juicer and process until juiced. Transfer to a serving glass and add some crushed ice before serving.

Enjoy!

**Nutritional information per serving:** Kcal: 147, Protein: 4.7g, Carbs: 46.8g, Fats: 1.1g

## 45.    Swiss Chard Juice

**Ingredients:**

2 cups of Swiss chard, chopped

1 cup of fresh kale, chopped

1 cup of collard greens, chopped

1 whole lemon, peeled

1 cup of cucumber, sliced

¼ tsp of ginger, ground

**Preparation:**

Combine Swiss chard, kale, and collard greens in a large colander. Wash thoroughly under cold running water. Slightly drain and roughly chop all. Set aside.

Peel the lemon and cut lengthwise in half. Set aside.

Wash the cucumber and cut into thin slices. Fill the measuring cup and reserve the rest in the refrigerator. Set aside.

Now, combine Swiss chard, kale, collard greens, lemon, and cucumber in a juicer. Process until juiced.

Transfer to a serving glass and stir in the ginger.

Serve cold.

**Nutritional information per serving:** Kcal: 57, Protein: 6.3g, Carbs: 17.8g, Fats: 1.2g

## 46.    Broccoli Brussels Sprout Juice

**Ingredients:**

1 cup of broccoli, chopped

1 cup of Brussels sprouts, halved

1 cup of cucumber, sliced

1 whole lime, peeled

¼ tsp of ginger, ground

**Preparation:**

Wash the broccoli and trim off the outer layers. Cut into small pieces and fill the measuring cup. Set aside.

Wash the Brussels sprouts and trim off the outer leaves. Cut each sprout in half and fill the measuring cup. Reserve the rest for in the refrigerator.

Wash the cucumber and cut into thin slices. Fill the measuring cup and reserve the rest for later. Set aside.

Peel the lime and cut lengthwise in half.

Now, combine broccoli, Brussels sprouts, cucumber, and lime in a juicer and process until juiced. Transfer to a serving glass and stir in the ginger.

Add few ice cubes and serve immediately.

**Nutritional information per serving:** Kcal: 63, Protein: 6.1g, Carbs: 19.5g, Fats: 1.2g

## 47.    Blackberry Avocado Juice

**Ingredients:**

2 cups of blackberries

1 cup of avocado, cubed

1 medium-sized apple, cored

¼ tsp of ginger, ground

**Preparation:**

Place the blackberries in a colander and wash thoroughly under cold running water. Slightly drain and set aside.

Peel the avocado and cut lengthwise in half. Remove the pit and cut into small cubes. Fill the measuring cup and reserve the rest in the refrigerator.

Wash the apple and cut in half. Remove the core and cut into bite-sized pieces. Set aside.

Now, combine blackberries, avocado, and apple in a juicer and process until juiced. Transfer to a serving glass and stir in the ginger.

Add some ice and serve immediately.

**Nutritional information per serving:** Kcal: 342, Protein: 7.7g, Carbs: 63.2g, Fats: 23.7g

## 48.   Raspberry Pear Juice

**Ingredients:**

1 cup of raspberries

1 large pear, chopped

1 whole lemon, peeled

1 small green apple, cored

**Preparation:**

Wash the raspberries thoroughly using a colander. Slightly drain and set aside.

Wash the pear and cut in half. Remove the core and cut into bite-sized pieces. Set aside.

Peel the lemon and cut lengthwise in half. Set aside.

Wash the apple and cut in half. Remove the core and cut into small pieces. Set aside.

Now, combine raspberries, pear, lemon, and apple in a juicer and process until juiced. Transfer to a serving glass and add some ice before serving.

Enjoy!

**Nutritional information per serving:** Kcal: 214, Protein: 3.6g, Carbs: 74.7g, Fats: 1.6g

## 49.    Coco Squash Juice

**Ingredients:**

1 cup of crookneck squash, sliced

1 medium-sized pear, chopped

1 cup of cucumber, sliced

1 whole lime, peeled

1 oz of coconut water

**Preparation:**

Peel the crookneck squash and scrape out the seeds with a spoon. Cut into small cubes and fill the measuring cup. Reserve the rest of the squash for some other recipe. Wrap in a plastic foil and refrigerate.

Wash the pear and cut in half. Remove the core and chop into small pieces. Set aside.

Wash the cucumber and cut into thin slices. Fill the measuring cup and reserve the rest in the refrigerator. Set aside.

Peel the lime and cut lengthwise in half. Set aside.

Now, combine squash, pear, cucumber, and lime in a juicer. Process until juiced. Transfer to a serving glass and stir in the coconut water.

Add some ice and serve immediately.

**Nutritional information per serving:** Kcal: 120, Protein: 2.4g, Carbs: 37.6g, Fats: 0.7g

## 50.   Kiwi Papaya Juice

**Ingredients:**

4 whole kiwis, peeled

2 small papaya, chopped

1 tbsp of fresh basil, roughly chopped

1 large banana, peeled

1 cup of cucumber, sliced

**Preparation:**

Peel the kiwis and cut in half. Set aside.

Peel the papaya and cut in half. Remove the seeds and dice into small pieces. Set aside.

Peel the banana and cut into chunks. Set aside.

Wash the cucumber and cut into thin slices. Fill the measuring cup and reserve the rest for later. Set aside.

Now, combine kiwis, papaya, basil, banana, and cucumber in a juicer and process until juiced. Transfer to a serving glass and add some ice before serving.

Enjoy!

**Nutritional information per serving:** Kcal: 365, Protein: 6.5g, Carbs: 107g, Fats: 2.8g

## 51.    Pepper Broccoli Juice

**Ingredients:**

1 large red bell pepper, chopped

1 cup of broccoli, chopped

1 cup of cucumber, sliced

1 large celery stalk, chopped

¼ tsp of ginger, ground

**Preparation:**

Wash the pepper and cut in half. Remove the seeds and stem. Cut into thin slices and set aside.

Wash the broccoli and trim off the outer wilted layers. Cut into small pieces and set aside.

Wash the cucumber and cut into thin slices. Fill the measuring cup and reserve the rest in the refrigerator.

Wash the celery stalk and cut into small pieces. Set aside.

Now, combine pepper, broccoli, cucumber, and celery in a juicer and process until well juiced. Transfer to a serving glass and stir in the ginger.

Refrigerate for 10 minutes before serving.

**Nutritional information per serving:** Kcal: 71, Protein: 4.9g, Carbs: 19.7g, Fats: 1g

## 52. Cantaloupe Orange Juice

**Ingredients:**

1 cup of cantaloupe, diced

1 small orange, peeled

1 cup of fresh mint, torn

1 whole lemon, peeled

¼ tsp of ginger, ground

**Preparation:**

Cut the cantaloupe in half. Scoop out the seeds and cut one medium wedge. Peel it and dice into small pieces. Reserve the rest of the cantaloupe in a refrigerator.

Peel the orange and divide into wedges. Cut each wedge in half and set aside.

Wash the mint thoroughly under cold water. Slightly drain and torn with hands. Set aside.

Peel the lemon and cut lengthwise in half. Set aside.

Now, combine cantaloupe, orange, mint, and lemon in a juicer and process until juiced. Transfer to a serving glass and stir in the ginger.

Add some ice before serving and enjoy!

**Nutritional information per serving:** Kcal: 104, Protein: 3.8g, Carbs: 33.2g, Fats: 0.8g

## 53.    Tomato Greens Juice

**Ingredients:**

7 cherry tomatoes, halved

2 cups of Swiss chard, torn

2 cups of collard greens, torn

1 cup of cucumber, sliced

1 whole leek, chopped

**Preparation:**

Wash the tomatoes and remove the stems. Cut each tomato in half and set aside.

Combine Swiss chard and collard greens in a large colander. Wash thoroughly under cold running water. Slightly drain and torn with hands. Set aside.

Wash the cucumber and cut into thin slices. Fill the measuring cup and reserve the rest for later.

Wash the leek and cut into small pieces. Set aside.

Now, combine tomatoes, Swiss chard, collard greens, cucumber, and leek in a juicer and process until juiced.

Transfer to a serving glass and refrigerate for 10 minutes before serving.

**Nutritional information per serving:** Kcal: 91, Protein: 6.2g, Carbs: 25.7g, Fats: 1.1g

## 54.    Mango Citrus Juice

**Ingredients:**

1 cup of mango, chunked

1 whole lemon, peeled

1 whole lime, peeled

1 small green apple, cored

1 tbsp of coconut water

¼ tsp of cinnamon, ground

**Preparation:**

Peel the mango and cut into small chunks. Fill the measuring cup and reserve the rest for later.

Peel the lemon and lime. Cut each fruit in half and set aside.

Wash the apple and cut in half. Remove the core and cut into bite-sized pieces. Set aside.

Now, combine mango, lemon, lime, and apple in a juicer and process until juiced. Transfer to a serving glass and stir in the coconut water and cinnamon.

Add some crushed ice and serve immediately.

**Nutritional information per serving:** Kcal: 178, Protein: 2.8g, Carbs: 53.4g, Fats: 1.1g

## 55.    Beet Kale Juice

**Ingredients:**

1 whole beet, sliced

1 cup of fresh kale, torn

1 small green apple, cored

1 small orange, peeled

¼ tsp of ginger, ground

**Preparation:**

Wash and trim off the beet. Slightly peel and cut into thin slices. Set aside.

Place the kale in a colander and wash under running water. Drain and torn with hands. Set aside.

Wash the apple and cut in half. Remove the core and cut into bite-sized pieces. Set aside.

Peel the orange and divide into wedges. Cut each wedge in half and set aside.

Now, combine beet, kale, apple, and orange in a juicer and process until juiced. Transfer to a serving glass and stir in the ginger.

Add some crushed ice and serve immediately.

**Nutritional information per serving:** Kcal: 153, Protein: 5.7g, Carbs: 44.6g, Fats: 1.1g

## 56.    Blueberry Kiwi Juice

**Ingredients:**

1 cup of blueberries

2 whole kiwis, peeled

1 whole lemon, peeled

1 cup of cantaloupe, diced

1 tbsp of coconut water

**Preparation:**

Place the blueberries in a colander. Wash thoroughly and drain. Set aside.

Peel the kiwis and lemon. Cut lengthwise in half and set aside.

Cut the cantaloupe in half. Scoop out the seeds and cut one large wedge. Peel it and cut into small pieces. Fill the measuring cup and reserve the rest of the cantaloupe in a refrigerator.

Now, combine blueberries, kiwis, lemon, and cantaloupe in a juicer and process until juiced. Transfer to a serving glass and stir in the coconut water.

Refrigerate for 10 minutes before serving.

**Nutritional information per serving:** Kcal: 196, Protein: 4.6g, Carbs: 59.8g, Fats: 1.6g

## 57. Cauliflower Spinach Juice

**Ingredients:**

5 cauliflower flowerets, chopped

1 cup of fresh spinach, torn

1 cup of pomegranate seeds

1 oz of water

¼ tsp of ginger, ground

**Preparation:**

Wash the cauliflower flowerets and chop into small pieces. Fill the measuring cup and reserve the rest for later.

Wash the spinach thoroughly under running water. Torn with hands and set aside.

Cut the top of the pomegranate fruit using a sharp paring knife. Slice down to each of the white membranes inside of the fruit. Pop the seeds into a measuring cup and set aside.

Now, combine cauliflower, spinach, and pomegranate in a juicer and process until juiced. Transfer to a serving glass and stir in the water and ginger.

Add some ice and serve immediately.

**Nutritional information per serving:** Kcal: 162, Protein: 3.1g, Carbs: 47,6g, Fats: 1.6g

# MEALS

## 1. GINGER MACKEREL & CUCUMBER SALAD

This amazing dish brings out the delicious taste and flavor of this ginger and cucumber combination. Ginger root is a powerful anti-inflammatory and anti-oxidant that acts by reducing the ability of tumors to grow. On the other hand, cucumber has lignans that have been shown to reduce the risk of uterine and prostate cancer.

**Ingredients:**

- 2 Mackerel fillets
- 1 Onion, chopped
- 1 Red pepper, chopped
- 1 lemon juice
- Fresh ginger, grated
- 1 garlic clove, minced
- 3 tbsp honey, separated 1-2
- 1 cucumber

- 2 tbsp dried wakame (seaweed)

- 4 tbsp Rice vinegar

- 1 tsp Sesame oil

- 1 tbsp Sesame seeds

- Salt and pepper to taste

**Instructions:**

✓ Rub the fish with salt and pepper;
✓ Prepare the marinade by mixing lemon juice, ginger and 1 tbsp honey, pour onto the fish and chill for about 30 minutes;
✓ Cut the cucumber into thin slices and sprinkle with salt, preserve for 10 minutes;
✓ Rehydrate the wakame by soaking in water as package instructions;
✓ Prepare the dressing mixing rice vinegar, sesame oil and remaining honey;
✓ Meanwhile, heat the grill and punt the fish skin side up on a baking sheet, grill for 5 minutes each side
✓ Wash and rinse the cucumber to remove the salt;
✓ Toss the cucumber and wakame together and sprinkle with sesame seeds;

✓ Serve the mackerel with the cucumber salad and spoon the dressing onto each serving.

## 2.    STUFFED PEPPERS

With this dish you will enjoy the perks of organic bell peppers, turmeric, garlic, onions and tomatoes, all filth with vitamins and compounds that boost your system and protect your body. For example, turmeric stimulates the apoptosis in cancer and reduces tumor growth, and tomatoes are a high source of Lycopene that also aids preventing growth cell of prostate cancer.

## Ingredients:

- 2 to 3 Colored bell peppers
- 1 cup Brown rice
- 1 tsp Cumin
- ½ tsp Turmeric
- 3 cups water
- Half Eggplant, chopped
- 1 Zucchini, chopped
- 1 Red Onion, diced
- 1 Garlic cloves, smashed
- 1 cup Natural tomato sauce

- 3 tbsp Olive oil

- Salt and pepper to taste

## Instructions:

✓ Preheat the oven to 380°F;

✓ Prepare de peppers: cut side up and remove seeds, scrub them inside-out with salt and pepper;

✓ In a saucepan boiled the water, rice, cumin, turmeric and a dash of salt, for about 12 to 15 minutes;

✓ Wash, peel and cut the eggplant, zucchini and onions into dices;

✓ In an oiled saucepan stir fry the vegetables until softened;

✓ When rice is ready, add it in batches to the vegetables, mixing between batches;

✓ Add the tomato sauce and mix well;

✓ Spoon filing into the prepared peppers, cover them with foil and bake for 20 minutes;

✓ Remove the foil and bake for 3 to 5 more minutes.

## 3.   RASPBERRY SALAD

This refreshing salad aims to care for your health, using the benefits of raspberries which contain ellagic acid, polyphenol and other compounds that promote the elimination of carcinogenic substances and inhibit angiogenesis.

## Ingredients:

- 4 cups Romaine Lettuce, sliced
- 2 cups Cress
- 2 cups Radicchio
- 2 cups Raspberries
- ¼ cup Almonds, chopped
- 6 tbsp Natural Pomegranate juice
- 3 tbsp Olive oil
- 3 tbsp Apple vinegar
- 2 tbsp Honey
- Salt and pepper to taste

## Instructions:

✓ Prepare the vinaigrette by mixing pomegranate juice, olive oil, apple vinegar, honey, salt and pepper, preserve;

✓ Wash and rinse the lettuce, cress and radicchio, cut roughly;

✓ In a big bowl put the green mixture and pour the vinaigrette on top and stir until combined;

✓ Sprinkle with almonds and serve.

## 4. FRUITY MORNING BOOSTER

Breakfast is the most important food of the day, this food will provide the energy to embrace your day full of energy while clean your body and revitalize your health. The incredible properties in these ingredients have shown to slow and prevent cancer development in color, liver, breast and prostate cells.

## Ingredients:

- 1 Ripe bananas, smashed
- 1 cup Whole wheat
- ¾ cup Almond milk
- 1 egg, slightly beaten
- 1 tsp Baking powder
- 1 tsp Baking soda
- 1 tsp Salt
- 2 tsp Vanilla
- ¼ cup Walnuts, chopped
- Preferred jam, fresh fruits or maple syrup.
- 1 cup hot water

- 2 tsp Green tea

- 1 tsp Ginger, minced

- Half lemon juice

- Honey to taste

**Instructions:**

For the tea:

✓ Put the tea and ginger into the hot water and set aside while making the pancakes;
✓ Then add the lemon juice and honey.

For the pancakes:

✓ Blend together almond milk, egg, banana, wheat, baking powder, baking soda, salt and vanilla;
✓ Coated a skillet with cooking spray and heat over medium;
✓ Pour ¼ cup batter onto the pan and sprinkle with walnuts, cook 1 minute each side;
✓ Serve with preferred jam, fresh fruits or maple syrup.

## 5.   DRIED TOMATOES FOCACCIA

This is a healthy meal option and a tasty treat. Keep enjoying the benefits of tomatoes, this time among whole-wheat, which is a great source of fiber. Dietary fiber is related with a lower risk some types of cancer, such as prostate, colon and colorectal cancer.

**Ingredients:**

- ¾ lukewarm water
- 2 tsp dry active yeast
- 1 tbsp honey
- 4 tbsp olive oil, divided
- 1 ½ cups whole wheat
- 1 tsp kosher salt
- 1 garlic clove, minced
- ½ cup dried tomatoes, chopped
- 1 tsp dried oregano

**Instructions:**

✓ Prepare a baking pan with baking spray;

✓ In a bowl combine water, yeast and honey, let it rest for 2 or 3 minutes;

✓ Add in the flour, garlic and oil, knead for 5 minutes;

✓ Spread the dough in the prepared pan and let it rise for 30 minutes;

✓ Once risen, preheat oven to 375°F;

✓ Sprinkle kosher salt, dried tomatoes and oregano over the dough and slightly press, drizzle with olive oil and bake for 10 minutes.

## 6.    FUNFETTI CABBAGE SLAW

Red cabbage is rich flavonoids that prevent the growth of precancerous cells that can lead to colon, colorectal and prostate cancer. In addition, carrots are loaded with beta-carotene, which are known for preventing a wide range of cancers, including prostate cancer.

**Ingredients:**

- 2 tbsp apple vinegar
- 1 tsp honey
- 1 tsp Dijon mustard
- 1 tsp poppy seeds
- 1 tsp olive oil
- Salt and pepper to taste
- 1 cup green cabbage, thinly sliced
- 1 cup red cabbage, thinly sliced
- ½ cup carrots, shredded
- ¼ cup brazil nuts, chopped

## Instructions:

✓ For the vinaigrette combine vinegar, honey, mustard, poppy seeds, olive oil, salt and pepper;

✓ Prepared the vegetables as described;

✓ Pour the vinaigrette onto the vegetables and toss;

✓ Sprinkle with brazil nuts and serve.

## 7.   HEALTHY CHILI

This chili is full of ingredients that are packed with nutrients: turmeric, onions, carrots, peppers, garlic, beans, and tomatoes! Everything in this mouthwatering plate is designed to improve your health. Even the simplest thing like garlic has amazing benefits with many anti-cancer effects. This organosulfur compounds like allicin and alliin triggers cell death in prostate cancer.

**Ingredients:**

- 1 tbsp oil
- Half onion chopped
- 2 bay leaves
- 1 tsp cumin
- ½ tsp turmeric
- 2 stalks celery, chopped
- 1 carrot, peeled and chopped
- 2 bell peppers, chopped
- 1 chili pepper, chopped
- 2 garlic cloves, minced

- 1 cup kidney beans, cooked and drained

- 1 cup black beans, cooked and drained

- 2 tomatoes, cooked, peeled and chopped

- 1 cup kernel corn

- 2 tbsp chili powder

- Salt to taste

- Freshly ground black pepper

**Instructions:**

✓ Prepare the ingredients as described;
✓ Heat the oil in a sauce pan and toss onions, bay leaves, cumin, turmeric and salt;
✓ Add in celery, peppers and garlic, and simmer for 5 minutes;
✓ Mix the tomatoes, chili powder, black pepper and all beans, let it boiled then simmer for 20 minutes;
✓ Toss the corn and combine, cook for 5 more minutes;
✓ Serve hot.

## 8.  MIGHTY BROCCOLI

Among the cruciferous, broccoli is well-known for preventing pre-cancerous cells from developing into malignant tumors; scientific studies demonstrated that it creates a strong defense against lung, prostate, breast, stomach, liver and ovarian cancer.

## Ingredients:

- Olive oil
- 2 garlic clove, minced and divided
- 1 tbsp ginger, minced
- 4 cups Broccoli florets
- 1 Onion
- 2 tbsp honey
- 1 tbsp apple vinegar
- Kosher salt to taste
- Fresh ground black pepper to taste

## Instructions:

- ✓ Preheat the oven to 400°F, prepare a baking pan coated with olive oil;
- ✓ Combine garlic, broccoli florets and salt, spread in the baking sheet and bake for 5 minutes
- ✓ Meanwhile, heat a skillet over medium with olive oil and sauté onions and a pinch of salt, until almost cooked;
- ✓ Add in garlic and ginger, stir over;
- ✓ Add honey and vinegar, low the heat;
- ✓ When ready, incorporate the broccoli and stir all together;
- ✓ Serve and enjoy.

## 9.    VEGGIE LASAGNA

This veggie lasagna is the perfect replacement for processed pasta, and it also provides the benefits of mushrooms, which contain polysaccharides and Lentinant, both anti-carcinogenic compounds.

## Ingredients:

- 1 tbsp olive oil
- 2 garlic cloves, minced
- 2 cups mushrooms
- 2 cups baby spinach
- 1 cup natural tomato sauce
- 2 to 3 zucchini, thinly sliced
- Salt and pepper to taste

## Instructions:

✓ Preheat the oven to 375°F;
✓ Heat the oil in a skillet and add in garlic, mushroom, salt and pepper, cook for a couple minutes;

- ✓ Incorporate baby spinach and tomato sauce, cook for 3 or 4 minutes;
- ✓ In a baking dish spoon some sauce at the bottom and arrange zucchini slices on top, repeat until all ingredients have been used;
- ✓ Bake for 20 minutes;
- ✓ Let it cool for a few minutes and serve.

## 10.   SAVORY PAPAYA SALAD

This exotic salad emphasizes the benefits of papayas, a rich fount of vitamin C and folic acid. This fruit has been shown to minimize absorption of cancer-causing nitrosamines from processed foods and prevent certain cancers, such as ovarian and prostate cancer.

## Ingredients:

- 1 garlic cloves, minced
- Kosher salt to taste
- 2 tbsp Wine vinegar
- 2 tbsp honey
- 2 tsp sriracha sauce
- 1 firm papaya, seeded and diced
- 1 red onion, sliced
- 1 tsp paprika
- Fresh ground black pepper to taste

## Instructions:

✓ Mix together papaya and onions

✓ In a medium bowl combine garlic, salt, vinegar, honey, sriracha sauce, paprika and ground pepper;

✓ Pour the mixture onto the papayas and onions and toss to incorporate;

✓ Serve and enjoy.

## 11. VEGGIE CURRY

Prepare to be pampered, with this veggie curry. You will absorb all the vitamins that you should to fight cancer. It will provide you with lots of lignans, flavonoids, beta-carotenes, lycopene, and more compounds that promise to take your health to another level and prevent you from getting a wide range of diseases.

**Ingredients:**

- Half onion, chopped

- 2 garlic cloves, smashed

- 1 tbsp ginger, grated

- ¼ dried tomatoes, chopped

- 1 tbsp olive oil

- 1 tsp cumin

- ½ tsp turmeric

- ½ tsp coriander

- 2 tbsp lentils

- 3 tbsp coconut milk

- 1 tbsp ground flaxseed

- ½ cup garbanzo beans, cooked and drained

- ½ cup pureed pumpkin

- Salt and pepper to taste

- Fresh coriander for sprinkle

## Instructions:

✓ Blend together onion, garlic, ginger, pumpkin and tomatoes until it resembles a puree.

✓ Heat oil in a saucepan and add in cumin, turmeric and coriander, then incorporate the puree mixture and let it boil;

✓ Lower the heat and add lentils and coconut cream, simmer for 5 minutes;

✓ Stir garbanzo beans and flaxseed and cook for 3 to 5 more minutes;

✓ Serve and sprinkle with fresh coriander.

## 12.    SAUCY SOUP

This saucy soup represents a new way to taste and harness the qualities of pumpkin and apples. On one hand, pumpkins are rich in carotenoids, lycopene and lutein, that increase the growth of immune cells and their capacity to attack tumor cells; on the other hand, apples are a good source of antioxidants and flavonoids.

### Ingredients:

- 3 cups pureed pumpkin
- 2 large red apples
- 2 tbsp olive oil
- 2 cups chicken broth
- ½ tsp cinnamon
- Salt and pepper to taste
- ¼ chopped brazil nuts, for sprinkle

### Instructions:

✓ In a skillet, heat oil and stir-fry diced apples with cinnamon, until apples start to caramelize;

✓ Incorporate pumpkin puree, then chicken broth, salt and pepper, cook for 7 minutes;

✓ Let it cool for a few minutes and blend together;

✓ Heat again if desired;

✓ Serve with Brazilian nuts sprinkled on top.

## 13.  GREEN TEA AVOCADO ICE-CREAM

This ice-cream it's full of vitamins, starting with an avocado base that is highly rich in antioxidants, aiding your system to attack free radicals. This innovative way of eating avocado by mixing it with matcha (a Japanese green tea powder) is definitely an enhanced way to enjoy ice cream.

**Ingredients:**

- 2 avocados, peeled and frozen
- ½ cup almond milk
- ½ cup coconut milk
- 2 tbsp matcha powder
- ¼ cup dates, chopped
- Dash ground cardamom

**Instructions:**

✓ Blend together almond milk, coconut milk, dates, cardamom and matcha powder, *add 1 to 2 tbsp honey if desired;

✓ Gradually incorporate frozen avocado until reached a creamy texture;
✓ Serve immediately or freeze overnight.

## 14. MATCHA MUFFIN DELIGHT

We've been talking about the benefits of green tea, matcha is an incredible form of green tea powder. To enjoy its benefits let's use it in dishes for creating healthy desserts like this one. This Japanese green tea powder is the richest source of polyphenols and catechins that are known for inhibiting metastases. Also, dark chocolate chips bring out the real flavor while providing a great source of antioxidants.

## Ingredients:

- 2/3 almond milk
- 2 tbsp cider vinegar
- 1 tbsp ground flaxseed
- 3 tbsp canola oil
- 1/3 honey
- Half banana, smashed
- 1 ½ whole wheat flour
- 2 tsp baking powder
- ½ tsp salt

- 2 tbsp matcha powder

- Dark chocolate chips *>70% cocoa

**Instructions:**

✓ Preheat the oven to 375°F and prepare a muffin pan;
✓ Combine almond milk, vinegar, and flaxseed, set aside for 5 minutes;
✓ Mix in oil, honey and banana;
✓ In a large bowl, combine flour, baking powder, salt and matcha powder;
✓ Pour liquid mixture into flour mixture and mix until almost combined (do not overmix);
✓ Add chocolate chips and slightly stir;
✓ Fill ¾ of the muffin pan with batter and bake for about 15 to 18 minutes.

## 15.   GREEN STUFFED MUSHROOMS

In this plate we combined the powerful properties of mushrooms, garlic, spinach, bell pepper and onion, but also we incorporated seaweed (wakame), which contain molecules that slow cancer growth in breast, colon and prostate cancers.

**Ingredients:**

- 2 large Portobello mushrooms caps
- 2 tbsp olive oil, divided
- 1 garlic clove
- 1 cup baby spinach
- 1 cup green bell pepper, diced
- 1 small onion, diced
- ½ dried wakame
- 1 to 2 tbsp oyster sauce
- Salt and pepper to taste
- Sesame seeds for sprinkle

## Instructions:

- ✓ Preheat oven to 400°F, slightly grease a baking pan;
- ✓ Rehydrate wakame as package instructions;
- ✓ In a large skillet heat the oil and stir fry bell pepper and onions until almost tender;
- ✓ Add spinach and garlic, sauté for a minute, and pour the oyster sauce, salt and pepper, cook for 3 to 4 more minutes;
- ✓ Remove from fire, stir rinsed wakame;
- ✓ Serve and sprinkle with sesame seeds.

## 16. SAUTEED SHRIMP & WHEAT-BERRY

Besides all the well-known benefits provided by broccoli, garlic, onion, scallions and endives, this recipe calls for wheat-berry, which contain wheat germ, thiamine, folate, zinc, and more compounds that ensure a balanced diet to prevent your system from any kind of disease.

**Ingredients:**

- 1 cup wheat berry
- 4 tbsp water
- 2 tbsp honey
- 2 tbsp rice vinegar
- 2 garlic clove, minced
- 2 cups broccoli florets
- 1 red onion, sliced
- 1 scallions, sliced
- 1 Belgian endive, sliced
- 2 cups raw shrimps
- 2 tbsp olive oil

- Salt and pepper to taste

## Instructions:

✓ Cook wheat berry as package instructions say, drain and let it cool;

✓ Meanwhile, whisk together water, honey, vinegar and garlic;

✓ Heat a skillet oiled and sauté the drained wheat-berry over high heat, stir constantly until crispy, preserve in a bowl;

✓ In the same skillet, sauté broccoli for a couple of minutes, add in onions and endives, salt and pepper, cook for 5 minutes;

✓ Incorporate shrimps and cook, add the wet mixture and stir for 2 minutes;

✓ Return wheat berry and toss until everything's combine;

✓ Serve and sprinkle with scallions.

## 17.    MIX QUINOA SALAD

The meal has a lot of phytochemicals, lycopene, lignans and allicin that not only prevent your system from diseases, but help to fight any carcinogenic cells, inhibiting them from spreading around our body. This dish also uses quinoa to provide a great amount of soluble fibers.

**Ingredients:**

- ¾ cup uncooked quinoa
- 1 cup natural chicken broth
- ½ cup dried tomatoes, chopped
- 1 garlic clove, smashed
- 2 cups kale
- 2 cups red cabbage
- 1 avocado, peeled, pitted and chopped
- 1 tbsp olive oil
- 1 tbsp balsamic vinegar
- 3 tbsp brazil nuts, chopped
- Salt and pepper to taste

## Instructions:

✓ Boil the broth and add in quinoa, salt and pepper, let it cook for 10 minutes, until the quinoa is tender and liquid is absorbed;

✓ In an oiled skillet quickly sauté garlic, kale, cabbage, salt and pepper, over high heat constantly stirring;

✓ Stir in quinoa and dried tomatoes, combine;

✓ Serve with avocados on top and drizzle with balsamic vinegar.

## 18.    GREEN SOUP KICK

Fully charge your system with this green soup, with vegetables packed with beta-carotene, glutathione, vitamins, and many antioxidants that will increase the production of protective enzymes that inhibit angiogenesis. Also, brazil nuts contain a lot of selenium, which has been linked with prostate cancer treatments.

## Ingredients:

- Half leek, sliced

- 1 garlic clove, minced

- 2 cups broccoli florets

- 2 cups asparagus, chopped

- 1 cup peas

- 5 cups natural vegetable or chicken broth

- 1 to 2 tsp sriracha sauce

- Half lemon juice

- Salt and fresh ground pepper to taste

- Chopped brazil nuts for sprinkle

## Instructions:

✓ Heat an oiled skillet and sauté leeks for 5 minutes, toss garlic and cook for one more minute;

✓ Add broth, broccoli florets, asparagus and peas, let it simmer for 7 minutes;

✓ Blend the soup and season with sriracha, lemon, salt and pepper;

✓ Serve and sprinkle with chopped brazil nuts.

## 19.    FRUITY BARS

Satisfy your cravings with these healthy fruity & nutty bars, rich in omega-3 fatty acids and many anti-carcinogenic agents found in peaches. On the other hand, pineapples are full of bromelain, an important component that fights cancer even better than the regular chemo drugs.

### Ingredients:

- 1 ½ cup almond flour
- 1 ½ cup oat flour
- ½ cup honey
- 2 tbsp canola oil
- 3 cups peaches, chopped
- 1 cup nectarines, chopped
- 1 cups pineapples, chopped
- 1 cups cherries
- ½ cup orange juice
- ½ cup pomegranate juice
- 2 tsp granulated jelly

## Instructions:

- ✓ Preheat the oven to 400°F and slightly grease a baking pan;
- ✓ Blend together almond flour, oat flour, honey and canola, until form clumps;
- ✓ Pour the mixture in to the baking pan and press down to form a layer, bake for 10 minutes or until golden brown;
- ✓ Meanwhile, prepare the filling heating an oiled saucepan to medium heat, stir in all the fruits and juice and simmer for 5 minutes;
- ✓ Mix the jelly with cold water;
- ✓ Remove the filling and cool for 5 minutes, incorporate hydrated jelly and stir until well combine;
- ✓ Pour the filling onto the baked crust and freeze over night;
- ✓ Cut the pie into bars and enjoy.

## 20.    BEST-HEALTHY TOMATO SAUCE

We bring the ultimate healthy tomato sauce to boost your body with the goodness of lycopene in tomatoes. This recipe is packed with different vegetables that provide a high source of fiber. Mixing them together is the best way to get the most from all the nutrients in them.

**Ingredients:**

- 3 tbsp Olive oil

- 3 cloves Garlic, minced

- 1 large Onion, diced

- 1 large Carrots, diced

- 1 Green pepper, diced

- 1 Zucchini, diced

- 1 cup Natural Chicken broth

- 2 pounds Tomatoes

- 2 tsp Paprika

- 3 tsp dried Oregano

- 3 dried Bay leaves

- 3 dried Basil leaves

- Salt and pepper to taste

**Instructions:**

✓ In a large saucepan heat oil and add paprika, oregano bay and basil leaves, stir for less than a minute and incorporate carrots and peppers, cook for 3 minutes and toss onions, garlic and zucchini, salt and pepper, cook for 8 to 10 minutes, after this, using tongs remove bay and basil leaves;

✓ Meanwhile, in another saucepan bring water to boil and add the tomatoes for 5 to 7 minutes, until the peel starts to rip, remove from heat and add cold water. When cold, finish peeling the tomatoes and drain the remaining water;

✓ When peeled, blend the tomatoes with chicken broth and pour into the vegetables, let it simmer for 20 minutes, stirring occasionally;

✓ If desired, you can blend all the ingredients to have an homogenic sauce, and add one or two anchovies' fillets to make the perfect sauce for a pizza.

## 21.   NO-KNEAD WHOLE WHEAT PIZZA DOUGH

Did you know there's a way to enjoy pizza and at the same time eat healthy? Because we all love to eat pizza, we want to show you a healthy pizza dough that can perfectly replace the processed pizza store. For enhanced taste and results, coat it with all natural tomato sauce, almond cheese (or other low fat cheese) and your favorite toppings.

### Ingredients:

- 3 cups whole wheat flour

- 1 tbsp instant dry yeast

- 1 tsp kosher salt

- 1 cup lukewarm water

- 1 tbsp olive oil

- 1 tbsp honey

### Instructions:

✓ In a large bowl combine dry ingredients;

✓ In a small bowl combine wet ingredients and pour it into the flour whilst stirring until incorporate and a shaggy dough forms;

✓ Transfer the dough into a clean and grease bowl and cover with plastic wrap, let it rest for 1 hour or until double it sizes;

✓ Gently deflate the dough using a wooden spoon, make two or three folders and let rest for 30 more minutes;

✓ When dough's ready, use a rolling pin to create a thin layer and cover with your favorites ingredients.

✓ Bake at 450°F for 10 to 13 minutes.

## 22.   RASPBERRY CRUMBLES

This decadent dessert has an incredible taste perfect to satisfy any craving for sweets, and also provides a high amount of nutrients and compounds beneficial towards the prevention of cancer. Such is the case of the ellagic acid found in raspberries, which stimulates apoptosis, being a natural anti-carcinogenic and anti-mutagen fruit.

### Ingredients:

- 2 cups raspberries
- 2 tbsp honey, divided
- 3 tbsp whole-wheat flour, divided
- 1 tbsp pomegranate juice
- ½ rolled oats
- ¼ cup chopped almonds
- ½ tsp cinnamon
- 1 tbsp canola oil

## Instructions:

✓ Preheat oven to 400°F;

✓ Combine raspberries, 1 tbsp honey, pomegranate juice and 1 tbsp flour, divided among 4 ramekins;

✓ Combine oats, almonds, cinnamon, remaining honey and flour, add oil and stir until just combine. Sprinkle over the fruit mix;

✓ Bake for 20 minutes, let it cool for 15 minutes before serving.

## 23.   MINI CALZONE

We want to teach you that been healthy doesn't mean you can't eat delicious food, so we bring this awesome mini calzone, a perfect treat for a family dinner while you stay on your nutritious diet.

## Ingredients:

- 1 ball homemade "No-Knead Whole-Wheat Pizza Dough"
- 1 cup Tomato sauce
- ½ cup Almond cheese
- ½ cup Fresh basil
- 1 cup Baby spinach
- Half Red onion
- ¼ cup Black olives
- 1 tsp Dried Oregano
- 1 tsp Dried Garlic
- 1 tsp Dried Thyme
- 1 tsp Red pepper flakes

- ½ tsp Ground black pepper

- 2 tbsp Olive oil

- 1 egg

## Instructions:

✓ Preheat oven to 400°F
✓ Cut the dough into 4 pieces, spread the pieces evenly in a floured surface to form 4 small pizzas;
✓ Toss all the filling ingredients together until combine;
✓ Spoon one or two tablespoon of filling mix on one half of each pizza and gently fold to form a half moon shape;
✓ Press the edges to seal;
✓ Coat with a beaten egg and sprinkle some kosher salt;
✓ Bake for 18 minutes.

## 24.    TUNA HEALTHY-PATTIES

For this plate we are focusing on the goodness of omega-3 fatty acids contained in tuna fillets, the anti-inflammatory and antioxidant properties of ginger, as well as olive oil, that provides more antioxidants and vitamins for your daily life.

**Ingredients:**

- 2 Tuna fillets, skinless
- 1 tbsp Curry paste
- 1 tbsp fresh ginger, grated
- 1 tbsp fresh dill, minced
- 1 tbsp fresh coriander, minced
- 1 tsp olive oil
- Salt and pepper to taste

**Ingredients:**

- ✓ In a food processor, blend tuna fillets, curry paste, ginger, dill, coriander, salt and pepper;

✓ Pour the mix into a bowl and shape into a burger;
✓ In an oiled skillet, fry the burgers for 4 minutes each side.
✓ Serve with whole wheat bread and preferred salad.

## 25.  SWEET & SPICY SALMON SUNSET

In this plate we combine sweetness and spiciness from mango and jalapeños, mangos are full of vitamins and beta-carotene compounds, while jalapeños are high in capsaicin that neutralize substance that might cause cancer.

**Ingredients:**

- 2 Salmon fillets
- 1 big mango, peeled and diced
- 1 red jalapeño, seeded and minced
- 1 fresh lemongrass, minced
- 1 tbsp rice vinegar
- 1 tbsp honey
- 2 tbsp olive oil, divided
- Salt and pepper to taste

**Ingredients:**

- ✓ Rub the fillets with salt and pepper;

✓ Combine mango, jalapeño, lemongrass, vinegar and honey;

✓ In a skillet heat 1 tablespoon of oil, place the salmon and cook for 3 minutes each side, set aside;

✓ In the same skillet heat the remaining oil and stir fry the mango mix for 3 or 4 minutes, add in the salmon and coat with juices and fruits;

✓ Remove from heat and serve;

## 26. FIG SALAD

Figs are awesome fruits for preventing and fighting cancer. Thanks to its derivatives of benzaldehyde, figs have been demonstrated to shrink tumors, and is also a great bacteria-killer.

### Ingredients:

- 4 figs, chopped
- 4 cups Romaine lettuce, chopped
- ½ Basil leaves
- ¼ Pecans, chopped
- 3 tbsp Cider vinegar
- 2 tbsp Fig relish
- 1 tbsp Olive oil
- Salt and pepper to taste

### Instructions:

✓ In a small bowl whisk together vinegar, relish, oil, salt and pepper;

✓ Toss the remaining ingredients in a large bowl;
✓ Pour dressing onto the green salad and combine;
✓ Serve with one piece of fig on top and sprinkle more chopped pecans.

## 27.   COLORFUL SKEWERS

Skewers represent a fun way of cooking and eating, and in this case these colorful skewers are filled with vitamins and beta-carotene found in bell peppers. Also it provides the benefits of bromelain from the pineapple, as mentioned before, this potent compound fights cancer and is more effective than chemo drugs.

## Ingredients:

- 1 Red pepper, chopped

- 1 Green pepper, chopped

- 1 Yellow pepper, chopped

- 1 Red onions, chopped

- 2 cups chopped Pineapples

- 2 tbsp Olive oil

- 1 Lemon juice

- 2 Garlic cloves, minced

- 1 tsp Paprika

- Salt and pepper to taste

## Instructions:

- ✓ Prepare all ingredients as described and thread them into the skewers alternating the ingredients;
- ✓ Whisk together lemon, garlic, paprika, oil, salt and pepper;
- ✓ Coat the skewers with the marinade and let them marinate for 30 minutes;
- ✓ Grill for 10 to 15 minutes.

## 28.   EASY GARLIC SOUP

As mentioned before, the anti-cancer benefits of garlic are many. Its immune-enhancing compounds aid the organism to fight and block carcinogenic cells, and studies have linked garlic to lower risk of stomach, colon and prostate cancer.

### Ingredients:

- 6 tbsp Olive oil
- 1 garlic head
- 2 tbsp whole-wheat flour
- 4 cups natural chicken broth
- Dried Thyme
- Dried Oregano
- Dried Basil
- Salt and pepper to taste

### Instructions:

✓ Cut garlic head in half -do not peel-;

✓ Heat an oiled saucepan to medium-low heat and place each half head flat, cook until garlic is soft and nicely browned, the peel will come out easily then;

✓ Remove from heat and smash the garlic with the flour combining well until a shaggy paste forms;

✓ Return to heat and add the hot broth, add thyme, oregano, basil, salt and pepper, cook until reached the desired consistency.

## 29.   TUNA SALAD

Once again we want to use the benefits of tuna and its omega-3 fatty acids, but this time combining the properties of radish, which are high in anthocyanins which are powerful anti-cancer molecules that prevent carcinogenic cells from developing.

**Ingredients:**

- 2 tune fillet, stir-fry
- 1 Red pepper
- 1 Red onion
- 2 Tomatoes
- 3 cups romaine lettuce
- 2 cups radicchio
- 1 cup radish, sliced
- 3 tbsp Greek Yoghurt
- 1 Lemon juice
- 2 tbsp Olive oil
- ½ tsp Mustard seeds, grounded

- Salt and pepper to taste

## Instructions:

✓ Whisk together yoghurt, oil, lemon, mustard seeds, salt and pepper;

✓ In a large bowl, combine peppers, onions, tomato, lettuce, radicchio and radish;

✓ Shred the tuna and stir it into the salad mixture;

✓ Drizzle with dressing and toss to incorporate.

## 30. BASIL ARUGULA PESTO

With this pesto you can create an awesome and healthy pizza or pasta, thanks to the essential oils in basil, which are part of the terpene family. They can promote apoptosis and reduce the spread of carcinogenic-cells.

### Ingredients:

- 4 cups fresh basil
- 1 ½ cup fresh arugula
- 3 garlic cloves
- ½ brazil nuts
- Half lemon juice
- ¼ tsp lemon zest
- 4 tbsp chicken broth
- ¼ cup olive oil
- Salt and pepper to taste

### Instructions:

✓ Pour all ingredients into a blender and blend until well mixed.

## 31.  HEALTHY SANDWICH

Alkaline foods such as alfalfa and avocado keep blood ph in its ideal range, which is very important for the prevention and treatment of cancer.

**Ingredients:**

- 4 slices Whole-wheat nutty bread
- 200gr Smoked salmon
- 1 cup Alfalfa
- 1 cup Watercress
- 1 Avocado, smashed
- 3 tbsp Greek yoghurt
- 2 tbsp Olive oil
- Salt and pepper

**Instructions:**

✓ Smash avocado and mix in yoghurt, oil, salt and pepper;
✓ Coat bread slices with avocado mixture;

✓ Arrange salmon, alfalfa and watercress, and cover with bread.

## 32.   JUICY CLEANSER

Fresh vegetable smoothies provide a valuable source of enzymes and antioxidant nutrients and are easily digestible. The well-known properties of pineapple, ginger, lemon and bee pollen makes this juice a perfect tonic for preventing cancer.

## Ingredients:

- 1 cup Water
- Half Cucumber
- 1 cup chopped Pineapples
- 1 stalk Celery
- 1 Lemon, juiced
- 1 tsp Ginger, grated
- 1 tsp Bee pollen
- 1 tbsp Honey
- 2 tbsp chopped Almonds

## Instructions:

- ✓ Rinse and peel fruits;
- ✓ Blend all ingredients together;
- ✓ Serve in a large glass and enjoy right away.

## ADDITIONAL TITLES FROM THIS AUTHOR

70 Effective Meal Recipes to Prevent and Solve Being Overweight: Burn Fat Fast by Using Proper Dieting and Smart Nutrition

By Joe Correa CSN

48 Acne Solving Meal Recipes: The Fast and Natural Path to Fixing Your Acne Problems in Less Than 10 Days!

By Joe Correa CSN

41 Alzheimer's Preventing Meal Recipes: Reduce or Eliminate Your Alzheimer's Condition in 30 Days or Less!

By Joe Correa CSN

70 Effective Breast Cancer Meal Recipes: Prevent and Fight Breast Cancer with Smart Nutrition and Powerful Foods

By Joe Correa CSN

www.ingramcontent.com/pod-product-compliance
Lightning Source LLC
Chambersburg PA
CBHW030247030426
42336CB00009B/287